Biomarkers used in Alzheimer's disease

Anay Mondal[1], Atul Kabra[*1]

[1]University Institute of Pharma Sciences, Chandigarh University, Panjab, India

Correspondence to: Dr. Atul Kabra, Associate Professor, Chandigarh University, NH05, Chandigarh-Ludhiana Highway, Gharuan, Mohali, Punjab -140413, India

Anay Mondal[1], Atul Kabra[*1]

Abstract:

Alzheimer's disease (AD) is a progressive neurological illness that significantly impairs memory, cognitive abilities, and day-to-day functioning. Timely and precise diagnosis is imperative for the effective management of the disease; however, existing clinical methodologies frequently fail to identify the disorder during its preclinical phase. Biomarkers, which may elucidate the underlying pathological mechanisms of AD, present considerable potential for earlier identification, enhanced diagnostic accuracy, and the monitoring of disease advancement. This review examines the most extensively researched biomarkers, which are classified into several categories: imaging biomarkers, cerebrospinal fluid (CSF) biomarkers, blood-based biomarkers, and genetic markers. Imaging techniques like magnetic resonance imaging (MRI) and positron emission tomography (PET) provide vital information about amyloid-beta buildup and neurodegenerative diseases. CSF biomarkers, notably amyloid-beta (Aβ42), tau, and phosphorylated tau (p-tau), serve as well-established indicators of AD pathology. Blood-based biomarkers are rapidly emerging as less invasive alternatives, bolstered by advancements in the detection of

Aβ, tau, and neurofilament light chain (NfL). Moreover, genetic markers, including the APOE ε4 allele, are explored concerning their association with susceptibility and the progression of the disease. The manuscript also addresses the obstacles encountered in biomarker development, emphasising the necessity for standardised testing protocols and longitudinal studies to evaluate their clinical relevance. Collectively, the incorporation of biomarkers into clinical practice holds the potential to transform the methodology for diagnosing and managing Alzheimer's disease, facilitating more individualised interventions and enhancing patient outcomes.

Keywords: Alzheimer's disease (AD), Biomarkers, Amyloid-beta (Aβ), Cerebrospinal fluid (CSF), Neurodegeneration, APOE ε4

Anay Mondal[1], Atul Kabra[*1]

Table of Contents:

Anay Mondal[1], Atul Kabra[*1]

1. Introduction:

Alzheimer's disease (AD) constitutes a neurodegenerative circumstance where cognitive abilities gradually deteriorate, memory dysfunction, & alterations in behaviour, thereby rendering it the predominant etiology of dementia. The affliction was initially delineated by Alois Alzheimer in 1906, subsequent to his identification of anomalous protein aggregates within the encephalon of a deceased individual exhibiting memory deficits and disorientation.

AD predominantly manifests in the geriatric population, with the majority of occurrences emerging post the age of 65, a phenomenon referred to as late-onset Alzheimer's disease (LOAD). A lesser fraction of instances, termed early-onset Alzheimer's disease (EOAD), arises within younger demographics and is frequently associated with genetic aberrations in genes such as APP, PSEN1, and PSEN2.

The progression of the disease transpires through a continuum, commencing with a preclinical phase wherein pathological alterations transpire years prior to the emergence of symptomatic manifestations, followed by mild cognitive impairment (MCI), & ultimately progressing to overt dementia. As reported by the World Health Organization (WHO), the prevalence of AD surpasses 50 million individuals globally, with projections indicating an escalation to 152 million by the year 2050. The rising incidence of AD, coupled with the absence of a curative intervention, poses a considerable public health challenge.

1.1 Importance of Biomarkers in Diagnosing, Predicting, and Monitoring AD

Biomarkers function as biological indicators that can be objectively quantified to evaluate physiological, pathological, or therapeutic responses to interventions. Within the context of Alzheimer's disease, biomarkers play a pivotal role in facilitating early diagnosis, tracking disease progression, and forecasting responses to therapeutic strategies.

Historically, the diagnosis of AD has predominantly depended on clinical evaluations, encompassing memory assessments and neuropsychological examinations, which were capable of confirming the disease predominantly in its advanced stages. The advent of biomarkers now facilitates the identification of AD-related neuropathological transformations during preclinical or early symptomatic phases, thus permitting earlier therapeutic intervention. For

Anay Mondal[1], Atul Kabra[*1]

example, cerebrospinal fluid (CSF) biomarkers such as amyloid-beta 42 (Aβ42) and tau proteins (including total tau and phosphorylated tau) can elucidate the pathological signatures of AD several years before the manifestation of cognitive symptoms. Likewise, positron emission tomography (PET) imaging targeting amyloid and tau proteins furnishes visual corroboration of AD pathology.

Blood-based biomarkers are also receiving increased scholarly interest due to their non-invasive characteristics and their potential applicability for extensive screening initiatives. These biomarkers, in conjunction with neuroimaging, are now incorporated into diagnostic frameworks, such as those formulated by the National Institute on Aging-Alzheimer's Association (NIA-AA) and the International Working Group (IWG).

Moreover, biomarkers are indispensable in the context of clinical trials, where they assist in the identification of suitable participants, monitoring therapeutic responses, and evaluating the efficacy of pharmacological interventions. They are also utilised for the stratification of patients based on the stage of the disease, thereby enabling tailored treatment approaches.

1.2 Current Challenges in Alzheimer's Disease Diagnosis and Treatment

Notwithstanding the progress achieved in biomarker research, substantial obstacles persist in the diagnostic and AD treatment landscape.

a. Early and Accurate Diagnosis:

A primary obstacle in the realm of Alzheimer's disease (AD) is the attainment of an early and precise diagnosis. Numerous patients receive a diagnosis only after the disease has advanced to a symptomatic phase, thereby constricting the opportunity for efficacious intervention. While biomarkers have enhanced early detection capabilities, their accessibility remains limited due to prohibitive costs, particularly concerning sophisticated neuroimaging modalities like positron emission tomography (PET). Furthermore, biomarkers such as cerebrospinal fluid (CSF), amyloid-beta (Aβ) and tau necessitate invasive lumbar puncture procedures, which constrains their application in standard clinical practice.

b. Lack of Effective Therapeutics:

The presently available therapeutic options for Alzheimer's disease, including cholinesterase inhibitors (e.g., donepezil) and NMDA receptor antagonists (e.g., memantine), offer

Anay Mondal[1], Atul Kabra[*1]

merely symptomatic alleviation without arresting or reversing the trajectory of disease progression. Although biomarker-driven pharmacological development has shown promise, a multitude of clinical trials targeting amyloid-beta and tau have failed to demonstrate significant clinical advantages. The controversial approval of aducanumab by the FDA in 2021, which targets amyloid, has prompted debate regarding its efficacy in enhancing cognitive outcomes.

c. Variability in Biomarker Expression:

Considerable heterogeneity exists in the pathological manifestation of AD among individuals, complicating the establishment of universally applicable biomarker thresholds. Certain patients may display elevated levels of amyloid plaques in the absence of cognitive deficits (designated as asymptomatic Alzheimer's disease), while others with analogous biomarker profiles may swiftly progress to dementia. This inherent variability complicates both diagnosis and prognostication, necessitating further investigative efforts to identify supplementary markers that can more accurately predict disease trajectory.

d. Ethical and Social Concerns:

Biomarkers used in Alzheimer's disease

The application of biomarkers for preclinical diagnosis engenders ethical dilemmas, particularly concerning the disclosure of biomarker findings to asymptomatic individuals. Receiving a diagnosis indicative of a preclinical stage of Alzheimer's disease can elicit considerable psychological distress and anxiety, especially in the absence of definitive therapeutic options. Additionally, it raises apprehensions regarding potential discrimination in employment and insurance based on genetic and biomarker data.

Anay Mondal[1], Atul Kabra[*1]

2. Pathophysiology of Alzheimer's Disease (AD)

The pathophysiological mechanisms underpinning AD are predominantly driven by the buildup of neurotoxic proteins within the cerebral environment, which disrupt neuronal functionality and ultimately culminate in cellular apoptosis. The two principal pathological hallmarks of AD are the intracellular aggregation of neurofibrillary tangles (NFTs), which are made of hyperphosphorylated tau protein, and the extracellular buildup of amyloid-beta (Aβ) plaques. The production of insoluble Aβ peptides that aggregate to form plaques results from the proteolytic cleavage of amyloid precursor protein (APP) by beta-secretase and gamma-secretase. These plaques interfere with synaptic transmission and precipitate a cascade of neurodegenerative processes. Hyperphosphorylated tau, a protein associated with microtubules, undergoes misfolding and aggregates into NFTs within neurons, disrupting axonal transport and culminating in cellular demise. In addition to protein aggregation, Alzheimer's disease is characterised by synaptic dysfunction, neuronal degeneration, gliosis, and cerebral atrophy, particularly within the hippocampus and cortex, regions that are pivotal for memory and cognitive functions. This multifaceted pathological landscape

12

underscores the complexity of AD and highlights formidable challenges related to its treatment and prevention.

2.1 Attribute of AD: Aβ Plaques and Tau Neurofibrillary Tangles

The defining characteristics of Alzheimer's disease encompass the presence of amyloid-beta (Aβ) plaques and tau neurofibrillary tangles (NFTs). Aβ plaques represent extracellular conglomerates of Aβ peptides that accumulate within the cerebral context as a consequence of aberrant cleavage of amyloid precursor protein (APP). These aggregates exhibit neurotoxicity, contributing to synaptic impairment, oxidative stress, and neuroinflammatory responses. The "amyloid hypothesis" posits that the aggregation of Aβ is an early and pivotal case in the pathogenesis of AD, engendering subsequent effects, including tau pathology. Conversely, tau protein typically serves to stabilise microtubules within neurons. In AD, tau undergoes hyperphosphorylation, resulting in its dissociation from microtubules and following assemblage into NFTs within neuronal cells. These neurofibrillary tangles disrupt normal cellular functionality, thus contributing to neurodegenerative processes. The "tau

Anay Mondal[1], Atul Kabra[*1]

hypothesis" posits a direct correlation between tau pathology and cognitive decline as well as neuronal demise. While both amyloid plaques and NFTs are regarded as fundamental features of AD, tau pathology demonstrates a more pronounced association with the severity and progression of the disease.

2.2 Role of Neuroinflammation and Oxidative Stress(OS) in AD Progression

In addition to the presence of $A\beta$ plaques and tau tangles, neuroinflammation and oxidative stress are instrumental factors in the progression of Alzheimer's disease. Neuroinflammation is instigated by the mobilisation of glial cells, notably microglia & astrocytes, in response to the deposition of amyloid. Despite their initial protective role, microglia's persistent activation exacerbates brain damage by releasing pro-inflammatory cytokines, reactive oxygen species (ROS), and other neurotoxic chemicals. Likewise, OS originates from an imbalance between the brain's antioxidant defences and ROS generation, which greatly contributes to cell death and neurological dysfunction. Both $A\beta$ plaques and tau pathology have been demonstrated to induce oxidative stress, thereby further accelerating synaptic impairment and mitochondrial dysfunction. The synergistic effects of chronic inflammation and oxidative stress engender a deleterious environment that exacerbates neurodegenerative trajectories, rendering them significant alleviative targets for mitigating the progression of AD.

Anay Mondal[1], Atul Kabra[*1]

3. Biomarkers

Biomarkers serve as quantifiable indices of biological activities, pathogenic mechanisms, or responses to therapeutic interventions. Within the framework of Alzheimer's disease, biomarkers furnish essential insights regarding the existence and advancement of disease pathology well in advance of the manifestation of clinical symptoms. They are indispensable for early diagnosis, monitoring the trajectory of the disorder, & assessing the effectiveness of curative modalities. Biomarkers can be identified within various biological fluids (e.g., cerebrospinal fluid (CSF), blood), or via imaging modalities and are increasingly utilised in clinical trials to enhance patient selection and monitor responses to experimental treatments. The establishment of dependable biomarkers for Alzheimer's disease is crucial for enhancing our comprehension of the disorder and improving clinical outcomes.

3.1 Types of Biomarkers:

Biomarkers pertinent to Alzheimer's disease can be comprehensively categorized into three distinct classifications: diagnostic, prognostic, and therapeutic response biomarkers.

Biomarkers used in Alzheimer's disease

Diagnostic biomarkers facilitate the identification of AD pathology, even in the void of overt cognitive symptoms. Prominent diagnostic biomarkers encompass diminished cerebrospinal fluid (CSF) levels of Aβ42 (which reflects amyloid plaque accumulation), elevated CSF tau levels (indicative of neurofibrillary tangles), and amyloid and tau positron emission tomography (PET) imaging.

Prognostic biomarkers yield insights regarding disease advancement and the probability of developing AD in individuals considered at risk. A pertinent example includes the APOE-ε4 allele status, which is a well-documented genetic susceptibility that heightens the likelihood of AD manifestation.

Therapeutic response biomarkers are employed to assess the effectiveness of therapeutic interventions through the measurement of alterations in relevant biomarkers. Such biomarkers are fundamental in determining whether a specific treatment is influencing disease-related biological mechanisms, such as the reduction of amyloid or tau accumulation or the mitigation of neuroinflammation. Each category of these biomarkers contributes uniquely to the comprehension and management of AD during the course of the disease.

Anay Mondal[1], Atul Kabra[*1]

4. Categories of Biomarkers in AD

Biomarkers associated with AD are critical instruments for the diagnosis of the disease, monitoring its progression, and assessing therapeutic strategies. These biomarkers are classified according to the particular pathological processes they represent, such as amyloid accumulation, tau pathology, neurodegeneration, neuroinflammation, and synaptic dysfunction, among others. The section that follows provides more details about the principal categories of biomarkers utilised in AD research and clinical practice.

4.1 Amyloid Biomarkers

Cerebrospinal Fluid (CSF) Amyloid-beta (Aβ) Levels

The evaluation of amyloid-beta (Aβ) concentrations in CSF constitutes one of the most established diagnostic modalities for the early identification of the pathophysiology of Alzheimer's. In the context of AD, CSF levels of Aβ42—a pivotal peptide implicated in amyloid plaque formation—are generally diminished as a consequence of its accumulation within the brain. The assessment of the Aβ42 to Aβ40 ratio, another isoform of amyloid-beta that does not accumulate in plaques, enhances diagnostic precision. The Aβ42/Aβ40 ratio is regarded as a more dependable marker

Anay Mondal[1], Atul Kabra[*1]

of amyloid pathology, as it accommodates individual variability in Aβ synthesis. This reduction in CSF Aβ42 is frequently observed several years prior to the emergence of cognitive symptoms, rendering it a valuable biomarker for early diagnosis and risk evaluation.

Amyloid PET Imaging

Amyloid positron emission tomography (PET) imaging represents a non-invasive modality that makes it possible to visualise amyloid plaques in the brain in vivo. Radiotracers like Pittsburgh Compound B (PiB) exhibit a specific affinity for amyloid plaques, allowing clinicians to detect and quantify amyloid deposition via PET scans. The advent of amyloid PET imaging has revolutionised the diagnostic landscape of AD, enabling researchers and clinicians to ascertain amyloid-positive individuals, even during the preclinical phases of the disease. This technique is particularly advantageous in clinical trials for confirming the presence of amyloid pathology and stratifying participants based on amyloid burden. Nonetheless, its elevated cost and restricted availability present significant barriers to widespread clinical implementation.

4.2 Tau Biomarkers
CSF Tau Levels

Biomarkers used in Alzheimer's disease

The accumulation of hyperphosphorylated tau protein inside the cerebral tissue is evidenced by an elevation in tau levels within the CSF. Two pivotal biomarkers indicative of tau pathology are total tau (t-Tau) and phosphorylated tau (p-Tau). t-Tau serves as a reflection of the cumulative burden of neuronal injury and degeneration, whereas p-Tau specifically denotes tau hyperphosphorylation and the resultant formation of neurofibrillary tangles, which are characteristic features of AD. Elevated concentrations of CSF p-Tau, particularly at designated phosphorylation sites (e.g., p-Tau181), exhibit a robust correlation with disease progression and cognitive decline, thereby establishing it as a critical biomarker for diagnosing and monitoring disease severity.

Tau PET Imaging

Analogous to amyloid PET, tau PET imaging facilitates the visualisation of neurofibrillary tangles within the cerebral context. Radiotracers such as [18F] flortaucipir exhibit selective binding to tau aggregates, thereby providing valuable insights into the spatial distribution and extent of tau pathology. Tau PET imaging is particularly instrumental in evaluating disease progression, as tau pathology generally displays a closer correlation with cognitive decline than

Anay Mondal[1], Atul Kabra[*1]

amyloid deposition. The capacity to image tau tangles in vivo has significantly advanced our comprehension of the mechanisms by which tau propagates throughout the brain and contributes to neurodegenerative processes.

4.3 Neurodegeneration Biomarkers

Neurofilament Light Chain (NfL)

When neurones are injured, a cytoskeletal protein called neurofilament light chain (NfL) is released into the circulation and cerebrospinal fluid. Elevated concentrations of NfL serve as indicators of neurodegeneration and are prevalent not only in AD but also in various other neurodegenerative disorders. NfL levels can be quantified in both CSF and blood, with blood-based assays providing a less invasive alternative for the detection of neurodegeneration. Enhanced NfL levels are associated with disease progression and may function as a biomarker for monitoring the efficacy of therapeutic interventions aimed at neurodegenerative processes.

Structural MRI

Magnetic resonance imaging (MRI) is extensively employed to evaluate cerebral atrophy, which is a defining characteristic of neurodegeneration in AD. Structural MRI quantifies alterations in brain volume, particularly within regions such as the hippocampus, which experiences notable atrophy in AD. Hippocampal atrophy exhibits a correlation with memory deficits and the severity of the disease, rendering MRI a valuable instrument for tracking disease progression. In addition to assessing hippocampal atrophy, whole-brain atrophy and cortical thinning can also be evaluated using MRI to monitor neurodegeneration longitudinally.

4.4 Neuroinflammation Biomarkers
Glial Fibrillary Acidic Protein (GFAP)

Glial fibrillary acidic protein (GFAP) acts as a biomarker for astrocyte activation, which transpires in response to neuroinflammatory processes. Augmented levels of GFAP in both CSF & blood have been documented in individuals diagnosed with AD, particularly during the advanced stages of the disease when neuroinflammatory mechanisms are more pronounced. GFAP has the potential to serve as a biomarker for the detection of astrocytic activation and inflammation associated with AD pathology.

CSF YKL-40

YKL-40 is classified as a glycoprotein that is secreted by activated microglia and astrocytes in the course of

Anay Mondal[1], Atul Kabra[*1]

neuroinflammatory responses. Raised levels of YKL-40 in the CSF are correlated with neuroinflammation and have been correlated with the progression of AD. The role of YKL-40 as a biomarker for identifying inflammatory responses in AD, as well as for differentiating AD from other neurodegenerative conditions, is currently under investigation.

TSPO PET Imaging

Translocator protein (TSPO) positron emission tomography (PET) imaging serves as a pivotal modality for visualising microglial activation within the cerebral context, thus providing a direct quantification of neuroinflammation. Radioligands, such as [11C]-PK11195, exhibit binding affinity to TSPO, a protein that is upregulated in activated microglia, thereby enabling researchers to delineate regions of neuroinflammation. The application of TSPO PET imaging is instrumental in elucidating the significance of inflammation in AD and in assessing the efficacy of anti-inflammatory therapeutic interventions.

4.5 Synaptic Dysfunction Biomarkers
CSF Synaptic Proteins

Synaptic dysfunction represents an early manifestation of AD and can be discerned through the analysis of synaptic proteins in cerebrospinal fluid (CSF). Proteins such as synaptotagmin and SNAP-25 are critical for facilitating synaptic transmission, and their concentrations in the CSF diminish concomitantly with synaptic loss in the context of AD. These proteins function as biomarkers indicative of early synaptic impairment, which precedes the more pronounced neurodegenerative processes.

Electroencephalography (EEG)

Electroencephalography (EEG) is a technique that quantifies electrical activity within the brain and is capable of detecting alterations in synaptic function that are associated with Alzheimer's disease. Variations in EEG waveforms, including diminished power in higher frequency bands alongside increased slow-wave activity, signify disturbances in neural networks that arise from synaptic degradation and neurodegeneration. EEG is a non-invasive modality that affords real-time insights into cerebral function and is currently being investigated as a possible biomarker for synaptic dysfunction in AD.

4.6 Blood-Based Biomarkers

Emerging Plasma Biomarkers (Aβ, Tau, NfL)

Anay Mondal[1], Atul Kabra[*1]

Recent advancements in the domain of blood-based biomarkers have facilitated the formulation of assays that can detect amyloid-beta, tau, and neurofilament light chain (NfL) in plasma samples. In addition to plasma phosphorylated tau and NfL, the plasma $A\beta42/A\beta40$ ratios are showing promise as non-invasive biomarkers for Alzheimer's disease diagnosis and tracking. These biomarkers have demonstrated robust correlations with their cerebrospinal fluid (CSF) equivalents and are more readily obtainable, rendering them advantageous for extensive screening and surveillance.

Proteomic and Genomic Approaches

Proteomic and genomic methodologies are being employed to unearth novel blood-based biomarkers pertinent to AD. Proteomic profiling facilitates the identification of protein signatures that correlate with the pathological features of Alzheimer's, whilst genomic investigations, including genome-wide association studies (GWAS), have recognised genetic risk factors (e.g., APOE-ε4) that contribute to the susceptibility to AD. These methodologies are augmenting our comprehension of AD and may lead to the identification of new biomarkers that facilitate early detection and personalised therapeutic strategies.

5. Genetic Biomarkers in AD

APOE-ε4 Genotype & Its Role in Risk Prediction

Among the most well-documented genetic susceptibility for AD is the presence of the APOE-ε4 allele. The APOE gene (apolipoprotein E) is integral to lipid metabolism & elimination of amyloid-beta (Aβ) from the cerebral matter. There exist three principal alleles of APOE: ε2, ε3, and ε4. The traces of the ε4 allele markedly heighten the risk of budding AD, with one possessing one copy of APOE-ε4 exhibiting a 3- to 4-fold elevation in risk, while those harbouring two copies manifest a 12- to 15-fold increased risk. Furthermore, the ε4 allele is correlated with an earlier onset of AD. The APOE-ε4 variant is postulated to hinder Aβ clearance, thereby fostering amyloid accumulation and plaque formation, in addition to contributing to synaptic dysfunction and tau pathology. Although APOE-ε4 is a potent predictor of risk, not all individuals with this allele advance to develop AD, indicating the influence of environmental factors and other genetic determinants.

Other Genetic Risk Factors (e.g., TREM2, PSEN1/2 Mutations)

Anay Mondal[1], Atul Kabra[*1]

Additionally to the APOE-ε4 allele, a multitude of other genetic variants have been linked to the susceptibility of Alzheimer's disease (AD). Mutations within the presenilin genes (PSEN1 and PSEN2) are correlated with the commencement of familial forms of AD. These PSEN1/2 mutations interfere with the functioning of amyloid precursor protein (APP), resulting in the augmented build-up of Aβ42, a notably fibrillogenic variant of amyloid-beta that tends to aggregate into plaques. Although these mutations represent a minor fraction of overall AD cases, they elucidate significant revelations about the molecular mechanisms that underpin the pathology of the disease. Another significant genetic contributor is TREM2 (triggering receptor expressed on myeloid cells 2), a gene responsible for regulating the functionality of microglia. Variants in TREM2 have been correlated with an elevated risk of AD due to their detrimental effect on the microglial capacity to eliminate amyloid plaques and respond effectively to neuronal damage. These genetic biomarkers provide substantial insights into the multifaceted biological pathways that contribute to the etiology of AD.

6. Multi-modal Biomarker Approaches

6.1 Combining CSF, Imaging, and Genetic Biomarkers

In efforts to enhance the precision of AD diagnosis & prognosis, multi-modal biomarker strategies amalgamate data derived from cerebrospinal fluid (CSF) biomarkers, neuroimaging techniques, and genetic profiling methodologies. For instance, amyloid PET imaging, which permits the visualisation of amyloid plaques, can be augmented by CSF assessments of Aβ42, thereby offering both structural and biochemical corroboration of amyloid pathology. Concurrently, tau PET imaging can elucidate the prevalence of tau tangles, while CSF levels of phosphorylated tau (p-Tau) provide comprehension into the biochemical status of tau hyperphosphorylation. The integration of genetic data, including APOE-ε4 status, facilitates the stratification of patients according to genetic risk, potentially pinpointing those individuals more predisposed to transition from mild cognitive impairment (MCI) to AD. The synthesis of these biomarkers affords a more holistic perspective of the disease trajectory, thereby enhancing diagnostic precision and enabling more accurate monitoring of disease advancement.

Anay Mondal[1], Atul Kabra[*1]

6.2 Integrating Machine Learning for Multi-modal Biomarker Analysis

Machine learning (ML) techniques are progressively being utilized for the analysis of multi-modal biomarkers in AD, thereby enabling the amalgamation of extensive and intricate datasets across various modalities. ML algorithms possess the capability to discern patterns within CSF biomarkers, neuroimaging data, and genetic information that might not be readily identifiable through conventional statistical methodologies. For instance, ML models can be developed to forecast disease progression by scrutinizing biomarker variations over time and detecting subtle trends that correlate with cognitive deterioration. Furthermore, these algorithms can facilitate patient stratification for clinical trials by identifying individuals at an elevated risk of disease progression based on comprehensive multi-modal biomarker profiles. The application of ML in the analysis of multi-modal biomarkers holds significant promise for advancing precision medicine in AD, allowing for earlier diagnosis and more tailored therapeutic interventions.

7. Role of Biomarkers in Disease Staging and Progression

7.1 Biomarkers for Early Detection and MCI Conversion to AD

A pivotal function of biomarkers in the context of AD pertains to the early identification of pathological changes preceding notable cognitive deficits. Cerebrospinal fluid (CSF) biomarkers, which include a diminished amount of Aβ42 and an elevated amount of phosphorylated tau (p-Tau), enable the detection of amyloid and tau pathologies during the preclinical phases of AD significantly before the manifestation of clinical manifestations. In patients diagnosed with mild cognitive impairment (MCI)—a critical intermediary stage linking normative ageing & AD—biomarkers can forecast progression to AD. The detection of amyloid positivity, ascertained via amyloid positron emission tomography (PET) or CSF Aβ42 quantification, augments the probability that individuals with MCI will transition to AD. Furthermore, biomarkers play an indispensable role in identifying subjects with prodromal AD, where minor cognitive impairments coexist with underlying AD pathologies.

Anay Mondal[1], Atul Kabra[*1]

7.2 Longitudinal Biomarker Changes Across Different Stages of AD

The longitudinal alterations in AD biomarkers are indicative of the disease's advancement through its various stages. In the initial phases, amyloid biomarkers, which include reduced CSF Aβ42 levels and positive amyloid PET findings, manifest first, frequently decades prior to the emergence of cognitive symptoms. As the disease evolves, tau biomarkers (for instance, elevated CSF p-Tau levels and tau PET imaging) become increasingly salient, correlating with the emergence of neurofibrillary tangles & cognitive deterioration. In the advanced phases, neurodegenerative biomarkers, like structural magnetic resonance imaging (MRI), revealing hippocampal atrophy & increased levels of neurofilament light chain (NfL) in CSF, signify extensive neuronal injury and loss. Monitoring these biomarker trajectories yields significant insights into the temporal succession of pathological incidents in AD, facilitating more accurate staging and a deeper comprehension of disease progression.

8. Clinical Utility of Alzheimer's Biomarkers

Use in Clinical Trials

Biomarkers have revolutionised the methodology involved in the design and implementation of clinical trials for AD. A fundamental application of biomarkers is in the enrichment of patient cohorts, wherein they are employed to select individuals exhibiting underlying AD pathology, even in the absence of overt clinical manifestations. For instance, individuals identified as amyloid-positive through PET imaging or CSF assessments are frequently recruited for trials evaluating anti-amyloid treatment modalities. Moreover, biomarkers are integral to monitoring disease progression and assessing therapeutic efficacy. Variations in amyloid PET or CSF tau concentrations can function as surrogate endpoints in clinical trials, providing indications regarding whether a therapeutic intervention is influencing the fundamental disease mechanism. This aspect has been particularly crucial in trials concerning disease-modifying therapies, where traditional cognitive assessments may require extended periods to become apparent.

FDA-Approved Biomarkers and Diagnostic Tools

Anay Mondal[1], Atul Kabra[*1]

In recent years, numerous AD biomarkers have attained approval from the Food and Drug Administration (FDA) for implementation in medical practice. Amyvid (florbetapir F18) has received FDA endorsement as a PET imaging agent for the identification of amyloid plaques within the cerebral context. Likewise, flortaucipir F18 has been sanctioned for tau PET imaging, facilitating the visualisation of neurofibrillary tangles. These imaging modalities are now employed within clinical environments to aid in the diagnosis of AD, particularly in scenarios where diagnostic clarity is lacking. Furthermore, advancements in blood-based biomarkers are progressing rapidly, with plasma p-Tau181 and NfL demonstrating potential as non-invasive diagnostic instruments. The FDA's endorsement of such biomarkers has broadened their clinical applicability, empowering clinicians to make more informed diagnostic and management decisions.

Biomarkers in Therapeutic Decision-Making and Patient Management

Biomarkers serve a pivotal function in the processes of therapeutic decision-making and patient management pertaining to AD. In light of the novel disease-modifying interventions that are presently emerging, such as anti-amyloid antibodies (for instance, aducanumab), biomarkers are employed to discern suitable candidates for treatment predicated on the identification of amyloid pathology. Furthermore, biomarkers are instrumental in the assessment of treatment efficacy, where decreases in amyloid PET signals or enhancements in cerebrospinal fluid (CSF) biomarker levels signify a favourable therapeutic result. Additionally, biomarkers are progressively incorporated into routine clinical practice to differentiate Alzheimer's from other etiologies of cognitive impairment, such as frontotemporal dementia or Lewy body dementia, thereby ensuring enhanced diagnostic accuracy and customised treatment strategies.

Anay Mondal[1], Atul Kabra[*1]

9. Emerging Biomarkers and Future Directions:

Novel Biomarkers Under Research (e.g., microRNA, Exosomes, Lipid Biomarkers)

Investigations into biomarkers for AD are increasingly extending beyond the conventional amyloid & tau markers, with microRNA (miRNA), exosomes, and lipid biomarkers surfacing as promising new research avenues. MicroRNAs, which are tiny non-coding RNAs that alter the expression of genes, have exhibited distinct expression profiles in AD patients in contrast to healthy controls. Specific miRNAs, including miR-29a and miR-107, are associated with pathways implicated in the production of amyloid-beta and tau phosphorylation, indicating their potential utility as diagnostic or prognostic biomarkers. Likewise, exosomes, which are diminutive vesicles including proteins, lipids, and nucleic acids secreted by cells, are under investigation as carriers of AD-associated proteins, such as amyloid-beta and tau, across the blood-brain barrier. Exosomal biomarkers may provide insights into the pathological processes occurring within the brain, offering a less invasive diagnostic approach for AD. Lipid biomarkers have also attracted scholarly attention, given the association of lipid dysregulation with the pathogenesis of AD. Lipidomic investigations have revealed alterations in sphingolipid, phospholipid, and cholesterol metabolism in patients with AD, which might be used as markers for early disease identification and disease progression assessment.

Challenges in Validating New Biomarkers

Despite the potential promise of novel biomarkers such as miRNAs, exosomes, and lipid profiles, their validation is fraught with numerous challenges. A significant concern is the inconsistency of findings across various studies, which may stem from disparities in methodologies, sample populations, and stages of the disease. The validation of biomarkers necessitates meticulous, large-scale studies encompassing diverse cohorts to guarantee reproducibility and generalizability. Moreover, the absence of standardised protocols for the collection, processing, and analysis of samples further complicates the validation endeavour. Another obstacle is the imperative for longitudinal studies to delineate the temporal relationship between novel biomarkers and disease progression, which is crucial for their clinical applicability.

Future trends: Liquid biopsies and point-of-care diagnostics

Anay Mondal[1], Atul Kabra[*1]

As the field advances, there is an increasing interest in liquid biopsies—minimally invasive assessments that identify AD biomarkers in body fluids like urine and blood. Blood-based assays targeting amyloid-beta, tau, and neurofilament light chain (NfL) have already shown significant correlations with their cerebrospinal fluid (CSF) equivalents. Liquid biopsies present the potential for early and widespread screening, as well as monitoring of disease progression, without the necessity for invasive procedures. Furthermore, technological advancements are facilitating the development of point-of-care diagnostics, wherein portable devices could yield real-time biomarker data within clinical environments. This development would enhance early detection, enable personalised treatment regimens, and allow for regular monitoring of disease progression in a more accessible manner.

10. Ethical Considerations and Limitations

10.1 Ethical Implications of Early Biomarker Testing

The capacity to identify biomarkers reflective of AD before the manifestation of clinical characteristics engenders a plethora of ethical dilemmas. A principal concern pertains to the ramifications of early biomarker testing on the psychological health of individuals. The awareness of being predisposed to developing Alzheimer's disease—potentially years preceding the emergence of symptoms—has the potential to precipitate anxiety, depressive disorders, and modifications in life choices, encompassing alterations in professional trajectories or family planning. Moreover, the informed consent process pertinent to biomarker testing necessitates that individuals comprehensively grasp the ramifications of the results, particularly in the context of the absence of efficacious disease-modifying interventions. Additionally, there exists the peril of genetic discrimination, wherein individuals recognised as possessing an elevated genetic susceptibility to Alzheimer's disease (e.g., carriers of the APOE-ε4 allele) may encounter obstacles in securing health insurance or employment, thereby highlighting the imperative for comprehensive legal safeguards.

Anay Mondal[1], Atul Kabra[*1]

10.2 The Psychosocial Impact of Biomarker-Based Diagnosis

A diagnosis of AD predicated on biomarker analysis, particularly during the initial stages or among asymptomatic individuals, can yield significant psychosocial repercussions. For individuals who have preclinical Alzheimer's disease or moderate cognitive impairment (MCI), the awareness of forthcoming cognitive deterioration can engender social isolation or stigmatisation. Patients and their families may endure amplified stress as they navigate the ambiguities associated with disease progression. The implications for caregiver burden represent another critical consideration, as caregivers frequently confront substantial emotional and financial adversities. To alleviate these consequences, healthcare practitioners must be equipped with methodologies that facilitate the provision of psychosocial support and promote transparent dialogue regarding the implications of biomarker findings.

10.3 Limitations in Accessibility, Cost, and Standardization of Biomarkers

Notwithstanding the rapid advancements in Alzheimer's disease biomarkers, significant limitations persist concerning their accessibility, financial implications, and standardization. Sophisticated biomarker assessments,

Biomarkers used in Alzheimer's disease

including PET imaging and cerebrospinal fluid analyses, are prohibitively expensive and not universally accessible, particularly in resource-constrained environments. The exorbitant costs associated with these procedures can engender disparities in diagnosis and treatment. Furthermore, the absence of standardization across laboratories and imaging facilities in the quantification of biomarker levels complicates the comparability of results across diverse studies or clinical environments. This variability accentuates the necessity for the harmonization of biomarker assays and the innovation of cost-effective, scalable diagnostic instruments to enhance the accessibility of biomarker testing.

Anay Mondal[1], Atul Kabra[*1]

11. Conclusion

In conclusion, biomarkers possess the capacity to fundamentally alter the paradigms of diagnosis, monitoring, and treatment modalities pertaining to Alzheimer's disease (AD). The evolution of imaging methodologies, cerebrospinal fluid examinations, and blood-based assays has enabled the identification of AD-associated pathologies at earlier stages, significantly preceding the manifestation of clinical symptoms. This critical early intervention period presents the opportunity to attenuate the progression of the disease and enhance patient outcomes; however, obstacles persist regarding accessibility, standardization, and ethical implications. Prospective avenues, such as the incorporation of multi-modal biomarker strategies and the application of machine learning techniques, exhibit considerable potential in tailoring AD management to individual patient profiles. Nevertheless, it is imperative to establish broader access, affordability, and ethical frameworks to facilitate the clinical utilization of biomarkers. Collectively, these initiatives contribute to the advancement of a more efficacious and equitable model for AD management, instilling optimism for improved patient care and therapeutic results.

www.ingramcontent.com/pod-product-compliance
Lightning Source LLC
Chambersburg PA
CBHW070140230526
45472CB00004B/1619